KETO MEA

Lose Weight, Save Time and Feel Your Best on the Ketogenic Diet

Annette Hubbell

Copyright © 2021.

All rights reserved to the author. No part of this book may be reproduced or transmitted via archive systems, file exchange systems, photocopies or others without the prior written authorization of the author.

Sommario

INTRODUCTION

Do you want to make a change in your life? Do you want to become a healthier person who can enjoy a new and improved life? Then, you are definitely in the right place. You are about to discover a wonderful and very healthy diet that has changed millions of lives. We are talking about the Ketogenic diet, a lifestyle that will mesmerize you and that will make you a new person in no time.

So, let's sit back, relax and find out more about the Ketogenic diet.

A keto diet is a low carb one. This is the first and one of the most important things you should now. During such a diet, your body makes ketones in your liver and these are used as energy.

Your body will produce less insulin and glucose and a state of ketosis is induced.

Ketosis is a natural process that appears when our food intake is lower than usual. The body will soon adapt to this state and therefore you will be able to lose weight in no time but you will also become healthier and your physical and mental performances will improve.

Your blood sugar levels will improve and you won't be predisposed to diabetes. Also, epilepsy and heart diseases can be prevented if you are on a Ketogenic diet. Your cholesterol will improve and you will feel amazing in no time.

How does that sound?

A Ketogenic diet is simple and easy to follow as long as you follow some simple rules. You don't need to make huge changes but there are some things you should know.

So, here goes!

MEAT

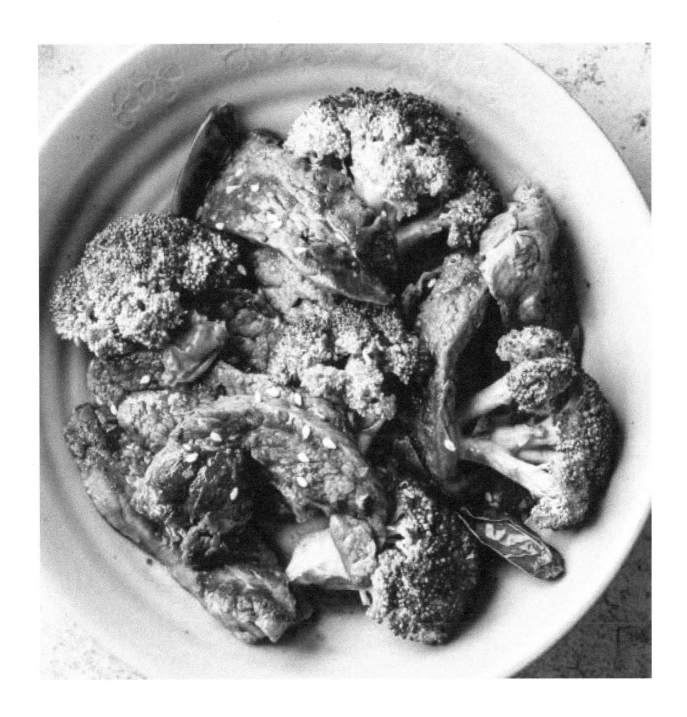

Moroccan Lamb

Try this Moroccan keto dish as soon as you can!

Preparation time: 10 minutes **Cooking time:** 15 minutes **Servings:** 4

Ingredients:

2 teaspoons paprika

2 garlic cloves, minced

2 teaspoons oregano, dried

2 tablespoons sumac

12 lamb cutlets

¼ cup olive oil

2 tablespoons water

2 teaspoons cumin, ground

4 carrots, sliced

¼ cup parsley, chopped

2 teaspoons harissa

1 tablespoon red wine vinegar

Salt and black pepper to the taste

2 tablespoons black olives, pitted and sliced

6 radishes, thinly sliced

Directions:

1. In a bowl, mix cutlets with paprika, garlic, oregano, sumac, salt, pepper, half of the oil and the water and rub well.

2. Put carrots in a pot, add water to cover, bring to a boil over medium high heat, cook for 2 minutes drain and put them in a salad bowl.

3. Add olives and radishes over carrots.

4. In another bowl, mix harissa with the rest of the oil, parsley,

cumin, vinegar and a splash of water and stir well.

5. Add this to carrots mix, season with salt and pepper and toss to coat.

6. Heat up a kitchen grill over medium high heat, add lamb cutlets, grill them for 3 minutes on each side and divide them between plates.

7. Add carrots salad on the side and serve.

Enjoy!

Nutrition: calories 245, fat 32, fiber 6, carbs 4, protein 34

Delicious Lamb And Mustard Sauce

It's so rich and flavored and it's ready in only half an hour!

Preparation time: 10 minutes **Cooking time:** 20 minutes **Servings:** 4

Ingredients:

2 tablespoons olive oil

1 tablespoon fresh rosemary, chopped

2 garlic cloves, minced

1 and ½ pounds lamb chops

Salt and black pepper to the taste

1 tablespoon shallot, chopped

2/3 cup heavy cream

½ cup beef stock

1 tablespoon mustard

2 teaspoons gluten free Worcestershire sauce

2 teaspoons lemon juice

1 teaspoon erythritol

2 tablespoons ghee

A spring of rosemary

A spring of thyme

Directions:

1. In a bowl, mix 1 tablespoon oil with garlic, salt, pepper and rosemary and whisk well.

2. Add lamb chops, toss to coat and leave aside for a few minutes.

3. Heat up a pan with the rest of the oil over medium high heat, add lamb chops, reduce heat to medium, cook them for 7 minutes, flip, cook them for 7 minutes more, transfer to a plate

and keep them warm.

4. Return pan to medium heat, add shallots, stir and cook for 3 minutes.

5. Add stock, stir and cook for 1 minute.

6. Add Worcestershire sauce, mustard, erythritol, cream, rosemary and thyme spring, stir and cook for 8 minutes.

7. Add lemon juice, salt, pepper and the ghee, discard rosemary and thyme, stir well and take off heat.

8. Divide lamb chops on plates, drizzle the sauce over them and serve.

Enjoy!

Nutrition: calories 435, fat 30, fiber 4, carbs 5, protein 32

Tasty Lamb Curry

This lamb curry is going to surprise you for sure!

Preparation time: 10 minutes **Cooking time:** 4 hours **Servings:** 6

Ingredients:

2 tablespoons ginger, grated

2 garlic cloves, minced

2 teaspoons cardamom

1 red onion, chopped

6 cloves

1 pound lamb meat, cubed

2 teaspoons cumin powder

1 teaspoon garama masala

½ teaspoon chili powder

1 teaspoon turmeric

2 teaspoons coriander, ground

1 pound spinach

14 ounces canned tomatoes, chopped

Directions:

1. In your slow cooker, mix lamb with spinach, tomatoes, ginger, garlic, onion, cardamom, cloves, cumin, garam masala, chili, turmeric and coriander, stir, cover and cook on High for 4 hours.

2. Uncover slow cooker, stir your chili, divide into bowls and serve.

Enjoy!

Nutrition: calories 160, fat 6, fiber 3, carbs 7, protein 20

Tasty Lamb Stew

Don't bother looking for a Ketogenic dinner idea! This is the perfect one!

Preparation time: 10 minutes **Cooking time:** 3 hours **Servings:** 4

Ingredients:

1 yellow onion, chopped

3 carrots, chopped

2 pounds lamb, cubed

1 tomato, chopped

1 garlic clove, minced

2 tablespoons ghee

1 cup beef stock

1 cup white wine

Salt and black pepper to the taste

2 rosemary springs

1 teaspoon thyme, chopped

Directions:

1. Heat up a Dutch oven over medium high heat, add oil and heat up.

2. Add lamb, salt and pepper, brown on all sides and transfer to a plate.

3. Add onion to the pot and cook for 2 minutes.

4. Add carrots, tomato, garlic, ghee, stick, wine, salt, pepper, rosemary and thyme, stir and cook for a couple of minutes.

5. Return lamb to pot, stir, reduce heat to medium low, cover and cook for 4 hours.

6. Discard rosemary springs, add more salt and pepper, stir, divide into bowls and serve.

Enjoy!

Nutrition: calories 700, fat 43, fiber 6, carbs 10, protein 67

Delicious Lamb Casserole

Serve this keto dish on a Sunday!

Preparation time: 10 minutes **Cooking time:** 1 hour and 40 minutes
Servings:

2

Ingredients:

2 garlic cloves, minced

1 red onion, chopped

1 tablespoon olive oil

1 celery stick, chopped

10 ounces lamb fillet, cut into medium pieces

Salt and black pepper to the taste

1 and ¼ cups lamb stock

2 carrots, chopped

½ tablespoon rosemary, chopped

1 leek, chopped

1 tablespoon mint sauce

1 teaspoon stevia

1 tablespoon tomato puree

½ cauliflower, florets separated

½ celeriac, chopped

2 tablespoons ghee

Directions:

1. Heat up a pot with the oil over medium heat, add garlic, onion and celery, stir and cook for 5 minutes.

2. Add lamb pieces, stir and cook for 3 minutes.

3. Add carrot, leek, rosemary, stock, tomato puree, mint sauce and stevia, stir, bring to a boil, cover and cook for 1 hour and

30 minutes.

4. Heat up a pot with water over medium heat, add celeriac, cover and simmer for 10 minutes.

5. Add cauliflower florets, cook for 15 minutes, drain everything and mix with salt, pepper and ghee.

6. Mash using a potato masher and divide mash between plates.

7. Add lamb and veggies mix on top and serve.

Enjoy!

Nutrition: calories 324, fat 4, fiber 5, carbs 8, protein 20

Amazing Lamb

This is a keto slow cooked lamb you will love for sure!

Preparation time: 10 minutes **Cooking time:** 8 hours **Servings:** 6

Ingredients:

2 pounds lamb leg

Salt and black pepper to the taste

1 tablespoon maple extract

2 tablespoons mustard

¼ cup olive oil

4 thyme spring

6 mint leaves

1 teaspoon garlic, minced

A pinch of rosemary, dried

Directions:

1. Put the oil in your slow cooker.

2. Add lamb, salt, pepper, maple extract, mustard, rosemary and garlic, rub well, cover and cook on Low for 7 hours.

3. Add mint and thyme and cook for 1 more hour.

4. Leave lamb to cool down a bit before slicing and serving with pan juices on top.

Enjoy!

Nutrition: calories 400, fat 34, fiber 1, carbs 3, protein 26

Lavender Lamb Chops

It's amazing and very flavored! Try it as soon as you can!

Preparation time: 10 minutes **Cooking time:** 25 minutes **Servings:** 4

Ingredients:

2 tablespoons rosemary, chopped

1 and ½ pounds lamb chops

Salt and black pepper to the taste

1 tablespoon lavender, chopped

2 garlic cloves, minced

3 red oranges, cut in halves

2 small pieces of orange peel

A drizzle of olive oil

1 teaspoon ghee

Directions:

1. In a bowl, mix lamb chops with salt, pepper, rosemary, lavender, garlic and orange peel, toss to coat and leave aside for a couple of hours.

2. Grease your kitchen grill with ghee, heat up over medium high heat, place lamb chops on it, cook for 3 minutes, flip, squeeze 1 orange half over them, cook for 3 minutes more, flip them again, cook them for 2 minutes and squeeze another orange half over them.

3. Place lamb chops on a plate and keep them warm for now..

4. Add remaining orange halves on preheated grill, cook them for 3 minutes, flip and cook them for another 3 minutes.

5. Divide lamb chops between plates, add orange halves on the side, drizzle some olive oil over them and serve.

Enjoy!

Nutrition: calories 250, fat 5, fiber 1, carbs 5, protein 8

Crusted Lamb Chops

This is easy to make and it will taste very good!

Preparation time: 10 minutes **Cooking time:** 15 minutes **Servings:** 4

Ingredients:

2 lamb racks, cut into chops

Salt and black pepper to the taste

3 tablespoons paprika

¾ cup cumin powder

1 teaspoon chili powder

Directions:

1. In a bowl, mix paprika with cumin, chili, salt and pepper and stir.

2. Add lamb chops and rub them well.

3. Heat up your grill over medium temperature, add lamb chops, cook for 5 minutes, flip and cook for 5 minutes more.

4. Flip them again, cook for 2 minutes and then for 2 minutes more on the other side again.

Enjoy!

Nutrition: calories 200, fat 5, fiber 2, carbs 4, protein 8

Lamb And Orange Dressing

You will love this dish!

Preparation time: 10 minutes **Cooking time:** 4 hours **Servings:** 4

Ingredients:

2 lamb shanks

Salt and black pepper to the taste

1 garlic head, peeled

4 tablespoons olive oil

Juice of ½ lemon

Zest from ½ lemon

½ teaspoon oregano, dried

Directions:

1. In your slow cooker, mix lamb with salt and pepper.

2. Add garlic, cover and cook on High for 4 hours.

3. Meanwhile, in a bowl, mix lemon juice with lemon zest, some salt and pepper, the olive oil and oregano and whisk very well.

4. Uncover your slow cooker, shred lamb meat and discard bone and divide between plates.

5. Drizzle the lemon dressing all over and serve.

Enjoy!

Nutrition: calories 160, fat 7, fiber 3, carbs 5, protein 12

Lamb Riblets And Tasty Mint Pesto

The pesto makes this keto dish really surprising and tasty!

Preparation time: 1 hour **Cooking time:** 2 hours **Servings:** 4

Ingredients:

1 cup parsley

1 cup mint

1 small yellow onion, roughly chopped

1/3 cup pistachios

1 teaspoon lemon zest

5 tablespoons avocado oil

Salt to the taste

2 pounds lamb riblets

½ onion, chopped

5 garlic cloves, minced

Juice from 1 orange

Directions:

1. In your food processor, mix parsley with mint, 1 small onion, pistachios, lemon zest, salt and avocado oil and blend very well.

2. Rub lamb with this mix, place in a bowl, cover and leave in the fridge for 1 hour.

3. Transfer lamb to a baking dish, add garlic and ½ onion to the dish as well, drizzle orange juice and bake in the oven at 250 degrees F for 2 hours.

4. Divide between plates and serve.

Enjoy!

Nutrition: calories 200, fat 4, fiber 1, carbs 5, protein 7

POULTRY

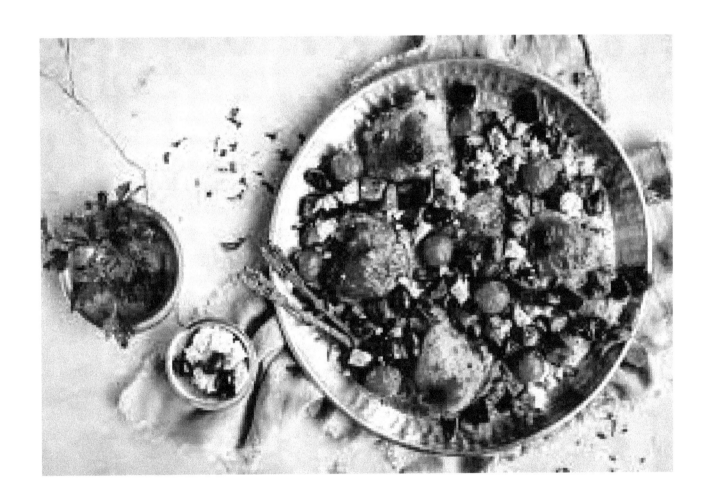

Unbelievable Chicken Dish

It's so yummy! We adore this dish and you will too!

Preparation time: 10 minutes **Cooking time:** 50 minutes **Servings:** 4

Ingredients:

3 pounds chicken breasts

2 ounces muenster cheese, cubed

2 ounces cream cheese

4 ounces cheddar cheese, cubed

2 ounces provolone cheese, cubed

1 zucchini, shredded

Salt and black pepper to the taste

1 teaspoon garlic, minced

½ cup bacon, cooked and crumbled

Directions:

1. Season zucchini with salt and pepper, leave aside few minutes, squeeze well and transfer to a bowl.

2. Add bacon, garlic, more salt and pepper, cream cheese, cheddar cheese, muenster cheese and provolone cheese and stir.

3. Cut slits into chicken breasts, season with salt and pepper and stuff with zucchini and cheese mix.

4. Place on a lined baking sheet, introduce in the oven at 400 degrees F and bake for 45 minutes.

5. Divide between plates and serve.

Enjoy!

Nutrition: calories 455, fat 20, fiber 0, carbs 2, protein 57

Delicious Crusted Chicken

You will soon end up recommending this amazing keto dish to everyone!

Preparation time: 10 minutes **Cooking time:** 35 minutes **Servings:** 4

Ingredients:

4 bacon slices, cooked and crumbled

4 chicken breasts, skinless and boneless

1 tablespoon water

½ cup avocado oil

1 egg, whisked

Salt and black pepper to the taste

1 cup asiago cheese, shredded

¼ teaspoon garlic powder

1 cup parmesan cheese, grated

Directions:

1. In a bowl, mix parmesan cheese with garlic, salt and pepper and stir.

2. Put whisked egg in another bowl and mix with the water.

3. Season chicken with salt and pepper and dip each piece into egg and then into cheese mix.

4. Heat up a pan with the oil over medium high heat, add chicken breasts, cook until they are golden on both sides and transfer to a baking pan.

5. Introduce in the oven at 350 degrees F and bake for 20 minutes.

6. Top chicken with bacon and asiago cheese, introduce in the oven, turn on broiler and broil for a couple of minutes.

7. Serve hot.

Enjoy!

Nutrition: calories 400, fat 22, fiber 1, carbs 1, protein 47

Cheesy Chicken

Your friends will ask for more!

Preparation time: 10 minutes **Cooking time:** 30 minutes **Servings:** 4

Ingredients:

1 zucchini, chopped

Salt and black pepper to the taste

1 teaspoon garlic powder

1 tablespoon avocado oil

2 chicken breasts, skinless and boneless and sliced

1 tomato, chopped

½ teaspoon oregano, dried

½ teaspoon basil, dried

½ cup mozzarella cheese, shredded

Directions:

1. Season chicken with salt, pepper and garlic powder.

2. Heat up a pan with the oil over medium heat, add chicken slices, brown on all sides and transfer them to a baking dish.

3. Heat up the pan again over medium heat, add zucchini, oregano, tomato, basil, salt and pepper, stir, cook for 2 minutes and pour over chicken.

4. Introduce in the oven at 325 degrees F and bake for 20 minutes.

5. Spread mozzarella over chicken, introduce in the oven again and bake for 5 minutes more.

6. Divide between plates and serve.

Enjoy!

Nutrition: calories 235, fat 4, fiber 1, carbs 2, protein 35

Orange Chicken

The combination is absolutely delicious!

Preparation time: 10 minutes **Cooking time:** 15 minutes **Servings:** 4

Ingredients:

2 pounds chicken thighs, skinless, boneless and cut into pieces

Salt and black pepper to the taste

3 tablespoons coconut oil

¼ cup coconut flour

For the sauce:

2 tablespoons fish sauce

1 and ½ teaspoons orange extract

1 tablespoon ginger, grated

¼ cup orange juice

2 teaspoons stevia

1 tablespoon orange zest

¼ teaspoon sesame seeds

2 tablespoons scallions, chopped

½ teaspoon coriander, ground

1 cup water

¼ teaspoon red pepper flakes

2 tablespoons gluten free soy sauce

Directions:

1. In a bowl, mix coconut flour and salt and pepper and stir.

2. Add chicken pieces and toss to coat well.

3. Heat up a pan with the oil over medium heat, add chicken, cook until they are golden on both sides and transfer to a bowl.

4. In your blender, mix orange juice with ginger, fish sauce, soy sauce, stevia, orange extract, water and coriander and blend

well.

5. Pour this into a pan and heat up over medium heat.

6. Add chicken, stir and cook for 2 minutes.

7. Add sesame seeds, orange zest, scallions and pepper flakes, stir cook for 2 minutes and take off heat.

8. Divide between plates and serve.

Enjoy!

Nutrition: calories 423, fat 20, fiber 5, carbs 6, protein 45

Chicken Pie

This pie is so delicious!

Preparation time: 10 minutes **Cooking time:** 45 minutes **Servings:** 4

Ingredients: ½ cup yellow onion, chopped

3 tablespoons ghee

½ cup carrots, chopped

3 garlic cloves, minced

Salt and black pepper to the taste

¾ cup heavy cream

½ cup chicken stock

12 ounces chicken, cubed

2 tablespoons Dijon mustard

¾ cup cheddar cheese, shredded

For the dough:

¾ cup almond flour

3 tablespoons cream cheese

1 and ½ cup mozzarella cheese, shredded

1 egg

1 teaspoon onion powder

1 teaspoon garlic powder

1 teaspoon Italian seasoning

Salt and black pepper to the taste

Directions:

1. Heat up a pan with the ghee over medium heat, add onion, carrots, garlic, salt and pepper, stir and cook for 5 minutes.

2. Add chicken, stir and cook for 3 minutes more.

3. Add heavy cream, stock, salt, pepper and mustard, stir and

cook for 7 minutes more.

4. Add cheddar cheese, stir well, take off heat and keep warm.

5. Meanwhile, in a bowl, mix mozzarella with cream cheese, stir and heat up in your microwave for 1 minute.

6. Add garlic powder, Italian seasoning, salt, pepper, onion powder, flour and egg and stir well.

7. Knead your dough very well, divide into 4 pieces and flatten each into a circle.

8. Divide chicken mix into 4 ramekins, top each with a dough circle, introduce in the oven at 375 degrees F for 25 minutes.

9. Serve your chicken pies warm.

Enjoy!

Nutrition: calories 600, fat 54, fiber 14, carbs 10, protein 45

Bacon Wrapped Chicken

The flavors will hypnotize you for sure!

Preparation time: 10 minutes **Cooking time:** 35 minutes **Servings:** 4

Ingredients:

1 tablespoon chives, chopped

8 ounces cream cheese

2 pounds chicken breasts, skinless and boneless

12 bacon slices

Salt and black pepper to the taste

Directions:

1. Heat up a pan over medium heat, add bacon, cook until it's half done, transfer to paper towels and drain grease.

2. In a bowl, mix cream cheese with salt, pepper and chives and stir.

3. Use a meat tenderizer to flatten chicken breasts well, divide cream cheese mix, roll them up and wrap each in a cooked bacon slice.

4. Arrange wrapped chicken breasts into a baking dish, introduce in the oven at 375 degrees F and bake for 30 minutes.

5. Divide between plates and serve.

Enjoy!

Nutrition: calories 700, fat 45, fiber 4, carbs 5, protein 45

So Delicious Chicken Wings

You will fall in love with this keto dish and you will make it over and over again!

Preparation time: 10 minutes **Cooking time:** 55 minutes **Servings:** 4

Ingredients:

3 pounds chicken wings

Salt and black pepper to the taste

3 tablespoons coconut aminos

2 teaspoons white vinegar

3 tablespoons rice vinegar

3 tablespoons stevia

¼ cup scallions, chopped

½ teaspoon xanthan gum

5 dried chilies, chopped

Directions:

1. Spread chicken wings on a lined baking sheet, season with salt and pepper, introduce in the oven at 375 degrees F and bake for 45 minutes.

2. Meanwhile, heat up a small pan over medium heat, add white vinegar, rice vinegar, coconut aminos, stevia, xanthan gum, scallions and chilies, stir well, bring to a boil, cook for 2 minutes and take off heat.

3. Dip chicken wings into this sauce, arrange them all on the baking sheet again and bake for 10 minutes more.

4. Serve them hot.

Enjoy!

Nutrition: calories 415, fat 23, fiber 3, carbs 2, protein 27

Chicken In Creamy Sauce

Trust us! This keto recipe is here to impress you!

Preparation time: 10 minutes **Cooking time:** 1 hour and 10 minutes
Servings:

4

Ingredients:

8 chicken thighs

Salt and black pepper to the taste

1 yellow onion, chopped

1 tablespoon coconut oil

4 bacon strips, chopped

4 garlic cloves, minced

10 ounces cremini mushrooms, halved

2 cups white chardonnay wine

1 cup whipping cream

A handful parsley, chopped

Directions:

1. Heat up a pan with the oil over medium heat, add bacon, stir, cook until it's crispy, take off heat and transfer to paper towels.

2. Heat up the pan with the bacon fat over medium heat, add chicken pieces, season them with salt and pepper, cook until they brown and also transfer to paper towels.

3. Heat up the pan again over medium heat, add onions, stir and cook for 6 minutes.

4. Add garlic, stir, cook for 1 minute and transfer next to bacon pieces.

5. Return pan to stove and heat up again over medium temperature.

6. Add mushrooms stir and cook them for 5 minutes.

7. Return chicken, bacon, garlic and onion to pan.

8. Add wine, stir, bring to a boil, reduce heat and simmer for 40 minutes.

9. Add parsley and cream, stir and cook for 10 minutes more.

10. Divide between plates and serve.

Enjoy!

Nutrition: calories 340, fat 10, fiber 7, carbs 4, protein 24

Delightful Chicken

It's a delicious and textured keto poultry dish!

Preparation time: 10 minutes **Cooking time:** 1 hour **Servings:** 4

Ingredients:

6 chicken breasts, skinless and boneless

Salt and black pepper to the taste

¼ cup jalapenos, chopped

5 bacon slices, chopped

8 ounces cream cheese

¼ cup yellow onion, chopped

½ cup mayonnaise

½ cup parmesan, grated

1 cup cheddar cheese, grated

For the topping:

2 ounces pork skins, crushed

4 tablespoons melted ghee

½ cup parmesan

Directions:

1. Arrange chicken breasts in a baking dish, season with salt and pepper, introduce in the oven at 425 degrees F and bake for 40 minutes.

2. Meanwhile, heat up a pan over medium heat, add bacon, stir, cook until it's crispy and transfer to a plate.

3. Heat up the pan again over medium heat, add onions, stir and cook for 4 minutes.

4. Take off heat, add bacon, jalapeno, cream cheese, mayo, cheddar cheese and ½ cup parm and stir well..

5. Spread this over chicken.

6. In a bowl, mix pork skin with ghee and ½ cup parm and stir.

7. Spread this over chicken as well, introduce in the oven and bake for 15 minutes more.

8. Serve hot.

Enjoy!

Nutrition: calories 340, fat 12, fiber 2, carbs 5, protein 20

Tasty Chicken And Sour Cream Sauce

You've got to learn how to make this tasty keto dish! It's so tasty!

Preparation time: 10 minutes **Cooking time:** 40 minutes **Servings:** 4

Ingredients:

4 chicken thighs

Salt and black pepper to the taste

1 teaspoon onion powder

¼ cup sour cream

2 tablespoons sweet paprika

Directions:

1. In a bowl, mix paprika with salt, pepper and onion powder and stir.

2. Season chicken pieces with this paprika mix, arrange them on a lined baking sheet and bake in the oven at 400 degrees F for 40 minutes.

3. Divide chicken on plates and leave aside for now.

4. Pour juices from the pan into a bowl and add sour cream.

5. Stir this sauce very well and drizzle over chicken.

Enjoy!

Nutrition: calories 384, fat 31, fiber 2, carbs 1, protein 33

FISH AND SEAFOOD

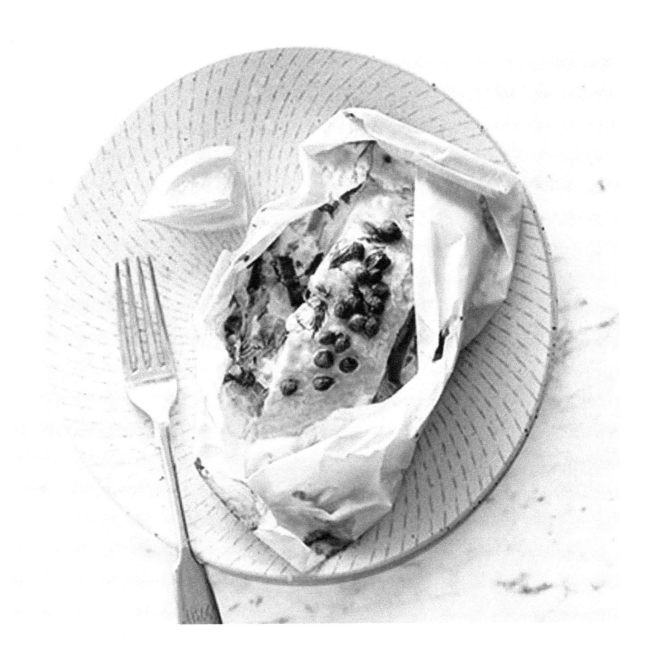

Cod Salad

It's always worth trying something new!

Preparation time: 2 hours and 10 minutes **Cooking time:** 20 minutes

Servings:

8

Ingredients:

2 cups jarred pimiento peppers, chopped

2 pounds salt cod

1 cup parsley, chopped

1 cup kalamata olives, pitted and chopped

6 tablespoons capers

¾ cup olive oil

Salt and black pepper to the taste

Juice from 2 lemons

4 garlic cloves, minced

2 celery ribs, chopped

½ teaspoon red chili flakes

1 escarole head, leaves separated

Directions:

1. Put cod in a pot, add water to cover, bring to a boil over medium heat, boil for 20 minutes, drain and cut into medium chunks.

2. Put cod in a salad bowl, add peppers, parsley, olives, capers, celery, garlic, lemon juice, salt, pepper, olive oil and chili flakes and toss to coat.

3. Arrange escarole leaves on a platter, add cod salad and serve. Enjoy!

Nutrition: calories 240, fat 4, fiber 2, carbs 6, protein 9

Sardines Salad

It's a rich and nutritious winter salad you have to try soon!

Preparation time: 10 minutes **Cooking time:** 0 minutes **Servings:** 1

Ingredients:

5 ounces canned sardines in oil

1 tablespoons lemon juice

1 small cucumber, chopped

½ tablespoon mustard

Salt and black pepper to the taste

Directions:

1. Drain sardines, put them in a bowl and mash using a fork.

2. Add salt, pepper, cucumber, lemon juice and mustard, stir well and serve cold.

Enjoy!

Nutrition: calories 200, fat 20, fiber 1, carbs 0, protein 20

Italian Clams Delight

It's a special Italian delight! Serve this amazing dish to your family!

Preparation time: 10 minutes **Cooking time:** 10 minutes **Servings:** 6

Ingredients: ½ cup ghee

36 clams, scrubbed

1 teaspoon red pepper flakes, crushed

1 teaspoon parsley, chopped

5 garlic cloves, minced

1 tablespoon oregano, dried

2 cups white wine

Directions:

1. Heat up a pan with the ghee over medium heat, add garlic, stir and cook for 1 minute.

2. Add parsley, oregano, wine and pepper flakes and stir well.

3. Add clams, stir, cover and cook for 10 minutes.

4. Discard unopened clams, ladle clams and their mix into bowls and serve.

Enjoy!

Nutrition: calories 224, fat 15, fiber 2, carbs 3, protein 4

Orange Glazed Salmon

You must try this soon! It's a delicious keto fish recipe!

Preparation time: 10 minutes **Cooking time:** 10 minutes **Servings:** 2
Ingredients:

2 lemons, sliced

1 pound wild salmon, skinless and cubed

¼ cup balsamic vinegar

¼ cup red orange juice

1 teaspoon coconut oil

1/3 cup orange marmalade, no sugar added

Directions:

1. Heat up a pot over medium heat, add vinegar, orange juice and marmalade, stir well, bring to a simmer for 1 minute, reduce temperature, cook until it thickens a bit and take off heat.

2. Arrange salmon and lemon slices on skewers and brush them on one side with the orange glaze.

3. Brush your kitchen grill with coconut oil and heat up over medium heat.

4. Place salmon kebabs on grill with glazed side down and cook for 4 minutes.

5. Flip kebabs, brush them with the rest of the orange glaze and cook for 4 minutes more.

6. Serve right away.

Enjoy!

Nutrition: calories 160, fat 3, fiber 2, carbs 1, protein 8

Delicious Tuna And Chimichurri Sauce

Who wouldn't love this keto dish?

Preparation time: 10 minutes **Cooking time:** 5 minutes **Servings:** 4

Ingredients:½ cup cilantro, chopped

1/3 cup olive oil

2 tablespoons olive oil

1 small red onion, chopped

3 tablespoon balsamic vinegar

2 tablespoons parsley, chopped

2 tablespoons basil, chopped

1 jalapeno pepper, chopped

1 pound sushi grade tuna steak

Salt and black pepper to the taste

1 teaspoon red pepper flakes

1 teaspoon thyme, chopped

A pinch of cayenne pepper

3 garlic cloves, minced

2 avocados, pitted, peeled and sliced

6 ounces baby arugula

Directions:

1. In a bowl, mix 1/3 cup oil with jalapeno, vinegar, onion, cilantro, basil, garlic, parsley, pepper flakes, thyme, cayenne, salt and pepper, whisk well and leave aside for now.

2. Heat up a pan with the rest of the oil over medium high heat, add tuna, season with salt and pepper, cook for 2 minutes on each side, transfer to a cutting board, leave aside to cool down a bit and slice.

3. Mix arugula with half of the chimichurri mix you've made and toss to coat.

4. Divide arugula on plates, top with tuna slices, drizzle the rest of the chimichurri sauce and serve with avocado slices on the side.

Enjoy!

Nutrition: calories 186, fat 3, fiber 1, carbs 4, protein 20

Salmon Bites And Chili Sauce

This is an amazing and super tasty combination!

Preparation time: 10 minutes **Cooking time:** 15 minutes **Servings:** 6

Ingredients:

1 and ¼ cups coconut, desiccated and unsweetened

1 pound salmon, cubed

1 egg

Salt and black pepper

1 tablespoon water

1/3 cup coconut flour

3 tablespoons coconut oil

For the sauce:

¼ teaspoon agar agar

3 garlic cloves, chopped

¾ cup water

4 Thai red chilies, chopped

¼ cup balsamic vinegar

½ cup stevia

A pinch of salt

Directions:

1. In a bowl, mix flour with salt and pepper and stir.

2. In another bowl, whisk egg and 1 tablespoon water.

3. Put the coconut in a third bowl.

4. Dip salmon cubes in flour, egg and then in coconut and place them on a plate.

5. Heat up a pan with the coconut oil over medium high heat, add salmon bites, cook for 3 minutes on each side and transfer them to paper towels.

6. Heat up a pan with ¾ cup water over high heat, sprinkle agar agar and bring to a boil.

7. Cook for 3 minutes and take off heat.

8. In your blender, mix garlic with chilies, vinegar, stevia and a pinch of salt and blend well.

9. Transfer this to a small pan and heat up over medium high heat.

10. Stir, add agar mix and cook for 3 minutes.

11. Serve your salmon bites with chili sauce on the side. Enjoy!

Nutrition: calories 50, fat 2, fiber 0, carbs 4, protein 2

Irish Clams

It's an excellent idea for your dinner!

Preparation time: 10 minutes **Cooking time:** 10 minutes **Servings:** 4

Ingredients:

2 pounds clams, scrubbed

3 ounces pancetta

1 tablespoon olive oil

3 tablespoons ghee

2 garlic cloves, minced

1 bottle infused cider

Salt and black pepper to the taste

Juice of ½ lemon

1 small green apple, chopped

2 thyme springs, chopped

Directions:

1. Heat up a pan with the oil over medium high heat, add pancetta, brown for 3 minutes and reduce temperature to medium

2. Add ghee, garlic, salt, pepper and shallot, stir and cook for 3 minutes.

3. Increase heat again, add cider, stir well and cook for 1 minute.

4. Add clams and thyme, cover pan and simmer for 5 minutes.

5. Discard unopened clams, add lemon juice and apple pieces, stir and divide into bowls.

6. Serve hot.

Enjoy!

Nutrition: calories 100, fat 2, fiber 1, carbs 1, protein 20

Seared Scallops And Roasted Grapes

A special occasion requires a special dish! Try these keto scallops!

Preparation time: 5 minutes **Cooking time:** 10 minutes **Servings:** 4

Ingredients:

1 pound scallops

3 tablespoons olive oil

1 shallot, chopped

3 garlic cloves, minced

2 cups spinach

1 cup chicken stock

1 romanesco lettuce head

1 and ½ cups red grapes, cut in halves

¼ cup walnuts, toasted and chopped

1 tablespoon ghee

Salt and black pepper to the taste

Directions:

1. Put romanesco in your food processor, blend and transfer to a bowl.

2. Heat up a pan with 2 tablespoons oil over medium high heat, add shallot and garlic, stir and cook for 1 minute.

3. Add romanesco, spinach and 1 cup stock, stir, cook for 3 minutes, blend using an immersion blender and take off heat.

4. Heat up another pan with 1 tablespoon oil and the ghee over medium high heat, add scallops, season with salt and pepper, cook for 2 minutes, flip and sear for 1 minute more.

5. Divide romanesco mix on plates, add scallops on the side, top with walnuts and grapes and serve.

Enjoy!

Nutrition: calories 300, fat 12, fiber 2, carbs 6, protein 20

Oysters And Pico De Gallo

It's flavored and very delicious!

Preparation time: 10 minutes **Cooking time:** 10 minutes **Servings:** 6
Ingredients:

18 oysters, scrubbed

A handful cilantro, chopped

2 tomatoes, chopped

1 jalapeno pepper, chopped

¼ cup red onion, finely chopped

Salt and black pepper to the taste

½ cup Monterey Jack cheese, shredded

2 limes, cut into wedges

Juice from 1 lime

Directions:

1. In a bowl, mix onion with jalapeno, cilantro, tomatoes, salt, pepper and lime juice and stir well.

2. Place oysters on preheated grill over medium high heat, cover grill and cook for 7 minutes until they open.

3. Transfer opened oysters to a heatproof dish and discard unopened ones.

4. Top oysters with cheese and introduce in preheated broiler for 1 minute.

5. Arrange oysters on a platter, top each with tomatoes mix you've made earlier and serve with lime wedges on the side. Enjoy!

Nutrition: calories 70, fat 2, fiber 0, carbs 1, protein 1

Grilled Squid And Tasty Guacamole

The squid combines perfectly with the delicious guacamole!

Preparation time: 10 minutes **Cooking time:** 10 minutes **Servings:** 2

Ingredients:

2 medium squids, tentacles separated and tubes scored lengthwise

A drizzle of olive oil

Juice from 1 lime

Salt and black pepper to the taste

For the guacamole:

2 avocados, pitted, peeled and chopped

Some coriander springs, chopped

2 red chilies, chopped

1 tomato, chopped

1 red onion, chopped

Juice from 2 limes

Directions:

1. Season squid and squid tentacles with salt, pepper, drizzle some olive oil and massage well.

2. Place on preheated grill over medium high heat score side down and cook for 2 minutes.

3. Flip and cook for 2 minutes more and transfer to a bowl.

4. Add juice from 1 lime, toss to coat and keep warm.

5. Put avocado in a bowl and mash using a fork.

6. Add coriander, chilies, tomato, onion and juice from 2 limes and stir well everything.

7. Divide squid on plates, top with guacamole and serve.

Enjoy!

Nutrition: calories 500, fat 43, fiber 6, carbs 7, protein 20

VEGETABLE

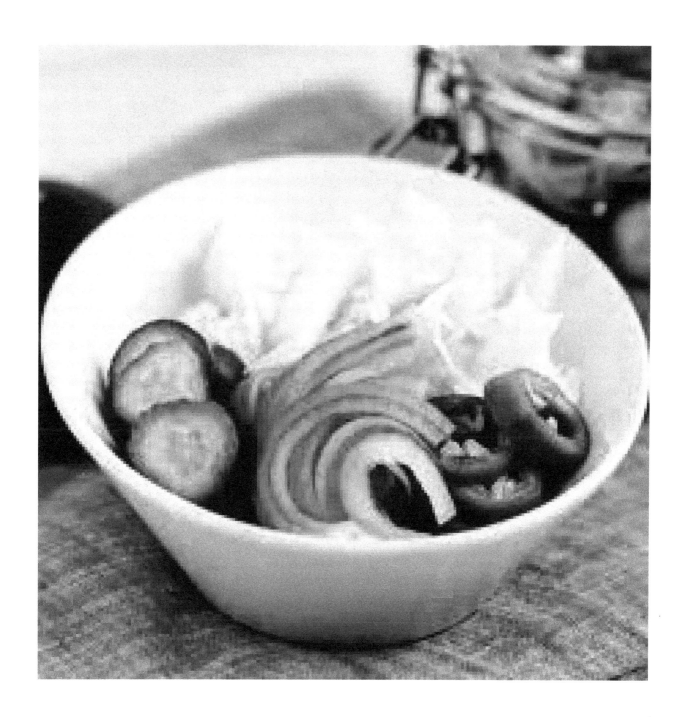

Avocado And Cucumber Salad

You will ask for more! It's such a tasty summer salad!

Preparation time: 10 minutes **Cooking time:** 0 minutes **Servings:** 4

Ingredients:

1 small red onion, sliced

1 cucumber, sliced

2 avocados, pitted, peeled and chopped

1 pound cherry tomatoes, halved

2 tablespoons olive oil

¼ cup cilantro, chopped

2 tablespoons lemon juice

Salt and black pepper to the taste

Directions:

1. In a large salad bowl, mix tomatoes with cucumber, onion and avocado and stir.

2. Add oil, salt, pepper and lemon juice and toss to coat well.

3. Serve cold with cilantro on top.

Enjoy!

Nutrition: calories 140, fat 4, fiber 2, carbs 4, protein 5

Delicious Avocado Soup

You will adore this special and delicious keto soup!

Preparation time: 10 minutes **Cooking time:** 10 minutes **Servings:** 4

Ingredients:

2 avocados, pitted, peeled and chopped

3 cups chicken stock

2 scallions, chopped

Salt and black pepper to the taste

2 tablespoons ghee

2/3 cup heavy cream

Directions:

1. Heat up a pot with the ghee over medium heat, add scallions, stir and cook for 2 minutes.

2. Add 2 and ½ cups stock, stir and simmer for 3 minutes.

3. In your blender, mix avocados with the rest of the stock, salt, pepper and heavy cream and pulse well.

4. Add this to the pot, stir well, cook for 2 minutes and season with more salt and pepper.

5. Stir well, ladle into soup bowls and serve.

Enjoy!

Nutrition: calories 332, fat 23, fiber 4, carbs 6, protein 6

Delicious Avocado And Bacon Soup

Have you ever heard about such a delicious keto soup? Then it's time you find out more about it!

Preparation time: 10 minutes **Cooking time:** 10 minutes **Servings:** 4

Ingredients:

2 avocados, pitted and cut in halves

4 cups chicken stock

1/3 cup cilantro, chopped

Juice of ½ lime

1 teaspoon garlic powder

½ pound bacon, cooked and chopped

Salt and black pepper to the taste

Directions:

1. Put stock in a pot and bring to a boil over medium high heat.

2. In your blender, mix avocados with garlic powder, cilantro, lime juice, salt and pepper and blend well.

3. Add this to stock and blend using an immersion blender.

4. Add bacon, more salt and pepper the taste, stir, cook for 3 minutes, ladle into soup bowls and serve.

Enjoy!

Nutrition: calories 300, fat 23, fiber 5, carbs 6, protein 17

Thai Avocado Soup

This is a great and exotic soup!

Preparation time: 10 minutes **Cooking time:** 10 minutes **Servings:** 4

Ingredients:

1 cup coconut milk

2 teaspoons Thai green curry paste

1 avocado, pitted, peeled and chopped

1 tablespoon cilantro, chopped

Salt and black pepper to the taste

2 cups veggie stock

Lime wedges for serving

Directions:

1. In your blender, mix avocado with salt, pepper, curry paste and coconut milk and pulse well.

2. Transfer this to a pot and heat up over medium heat.

3. Add stock, stir, bring to a simmer and cook for 5 minutes.

4. Add cilantro, more salt and pepper, stir, cook for 1 minute more, ladle into soup bowls and serve with lime wedges on the side.

Enjoy!

Nutrition: calories 240, fat 4, fiber 2, carbs 6, protein 12

Simple Arugula Salad

It's light and very tasty! Try it for dinner!

Preparation time: 10 minutes **Cooking time:** 0 minutes **Servings:** 4

Ingredients:

1 white onion, chopped

1 tablespoon vinegar

1 cup hot water

1 bunch baby arugula

¼ cup walnuts, chopped

2 tablespoons cilantro, chopped

2 garlic cloves, minced

2 tablespoons olive oil

Salt and black pepper to the taste

1 tablespoon lemon juice

Directions:

1. In a bowl, mix water with vinegar, add onion, leave aside for 5 minutes, drain well and press.

2. In a salad bowl, mix arugula with walnuts and onion and stir.

3. Add garlic, salt, pepper, lemon juice, cilantro and oil, toss well and serve.

Enjoy!

Nutrition: calories 200, fat 2, fiber 1, carbs 5, protein 7

Arugula Soup

You have to try this great keto soup as soon as you can!

Preparation time: 10 minutes **Cooking time:** 13 minutes **Servings:** 6

Ingredients:

1 yellow onion, chopped

1 tablespoon olive oil

2 garlic cloves, minced

½ cup coconut milk

10 ounces baby arugula

¼ cup mixed mint, tarragon and parsley

2 tablespoons chives, chopped

4 tablespoons coconut milk yogurt

6 cups chicken stock

Salt and black pepper to the taste

Directions:

1. Heat up a pot with the oil over medium high heat, add onion and garlic, stir and cook for 5 minutes.

2. Add stock and milk, stir and bring to a simmer.

3. Add arugula, tarragon, parsley and mint, stir and cook everything for 6 minutes.

4. Add coconut yogurt, salt, pepper and chives, stir, cook for 2 minutes, divide into soup bowls and serve.

Enjoy!

Nutrition: calories 200, fat 4, fiber 2, carbs 6, protein 10

Arugula And Broccoli Soup

It's one of our favorite soups!

Preparation time: 10 minutes **Cooking time:** 20 minutes **Servings:** 4

Ingredients:

1 small yellow onion, chopped

1 tablespoon olive oil

1 garlic clove, minced

1 broccoli head, florets separated

Salt and black pepper to the taste

2 and ½ cups veggie stock

1 teaspoon cumin, ground

Juice of ½ lemon

1 cup arugula leaves

Directions:

1. Heat up a pot with the oil over medium high heat, add onions, stir and cook for 4 minutes.

2. Add garlic, stir and cook for 1 minute.

3. Add broccoli, cumin, salt and pepper, stir and cook for 4 minutes.

4. Add stock, stir and cook for 8 minutes.

5. Blend soup using an immersion blender, add half of the arugula and blend again.

6. Add the rest of the arugula, stir and heat up the soup again.

7. Add lemon juice, stir, ladle into soup bowls and serve.

Enjoy!

Nutrition: calories 150, fat 3, fiber 1, carbs 3, protein 7

Delicious Zucchini Cream

This is a keto comfort food you will enjoy for sure!

Preparation time: 10 minutes **Cooking time:** 25 minutes **Servings:** 8

Ingredients:

6 zucchinis, cut in halves and then sliced

Salt and black pepper to the taste

1 tablespoon ghee

28 ounces veggie stock

1 teaspoon oregano, dried

½ cup yellow onion, chopped

3 garlic cloves, minced

2 ounces parmesan, grated

¾ cup heavy cream

Directions:

1. Heat up a pot with the ghee over medium high heat, add onion, stir and cook for 4 minutes.

2. Add garlic, stir and cook for 2 minutes more.

3. Add zucchinis, stir and cook for 3 minutes.

4. Add stock, stir, bring to a boil and simmer over medium heat for 15 minutes.

5. Add oregano, salt and pepper, stir, take off heat and blend using an immersion blender.

6. Heat up soup again, add heavy cream, stir and bring to a simmer.

7. Add parmesan, stir, take off heat, ladle into bowls and serve right away.

Enjoy!

Nutrition: calories 160, fat 4, fiber 2, carbs 4, protein 8

Zucchini And Avocado Soup

This keto soup is full of tasty ingredient and healthy elements!

Preparation time: 10 minutes **Cooking time:** 15 minutes **Servings:** 4

Ingredients:

1 big avocado, pitted, peeled and chopped

4 scallions, chopped

1 teaspoon ginger, grated

2 tablespoons avocado oil

Salt and black pepper to the taste

2 zucchinis, chopped

29 ounces veggie stock

1 garlic clove, minced

1 cup water

1 tablespoon lemon juice

1 red bell pepper, chopped

Directions:

1. Heat up a pot with the oil over medium heat, add onions, stir and cook for 3 minutes.

2. Add garlic and ginger, stir and cook for 1 minute.

3. Add zucchini, salt, pepper, water and stock, stir, bring to a boil, cover pot and cook for 10 minutes.

4. Take off heat, leave soup aside for a couple of minutes, add avocado, stir, blend everything using an immersion blender and heat up again.

5. Add more salt and pepper, bell pepper and lemon juice, stir, heat up soup again, ladle into soup bowls and serve.

Enjoy!

Nutrition: calories 154, fat 12, fiber 3, carbs 5, protein 4

Swiss Chard Pie

You will always remember this amazing taste!

Preparation time: 10 minutes **Cooking time:** 45 minutes **Servings:** 12

Ingredients:

8 cups Swiss chard, chopped

½ cup onion, chopped

1 tablespoon olive oil

1 garlic clove, minced

Salt and black pepper to the taste

3 eggs

2 cups ricotta cheese

1 cup mozzarella, shredded

A pinch of nutmeg

¼ cup parmesan, grated

1 pound sausage, chopped

Directions:

1. Heat up a pan with the oil over medium heat, add onions and garlic, stir and cook for 3 minutes.

2. Add Swiss chard, stir and cook for 5 minutes more.

3. Add salt, pepper and nutmeg, stir, take off heat and leave aside for a few minutes.

4. In a bowl, whisk eggs with mozzarella, parmesan and ricotta and stir well.

5. Add Swiss chard mix and stir well.

6. Spread sausage meat on the bottom of a pie pan and press well.

7. Add Swiss chard and eggs mix, spread well, introduce in the oven at 350 degrees F and bake for 35 minutes.

8. Leave pie aside to cool down, slice and serve it.

Enjoy!

Nutrition: calories 332, fat 23, fiber 3, carbs 4, protein 23

DESSERT

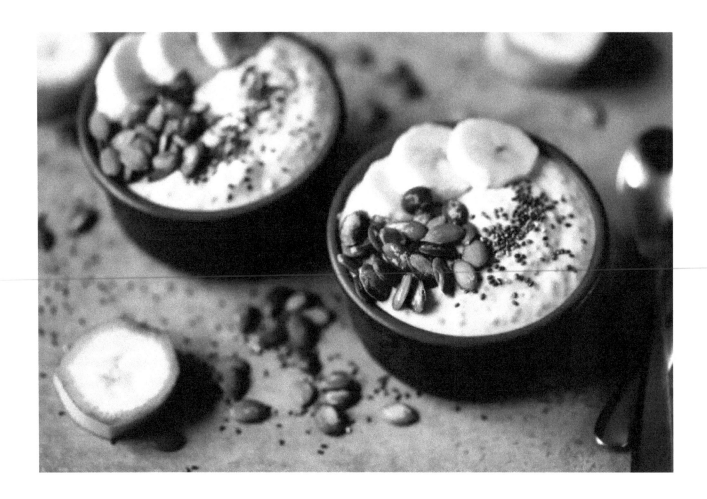

Amazing Peanut Butter And Chia Pudding

The combination is very delicious!

Preparation time: 10 minutes **Cooking time:** 0 minutes **Servings:** 4

Ingredients: ½ cup chia seeds

2 cups almond milk, unsweetened

1 teaspoon vanilla extract

¼ cup peanut butter, unsweetened

1 teaspoon vanilla stevia

A pinch of salt

Directions:

1. In a bowl, mix milk with chia seeds, peanut butter, vanilla extract, stevia and pinch of salt and stir well.

2. Leave this pudding aside for 5 minutes, then stir it again, divide into dessert glasses and leave in the fridge for 10 minutes.

Enjoy!

Nutrition: calories 120, fat 1, fiber 2, carbs 4, protein 2

Tasty Pumpkin Custard

It's one of our favorite keto desserts! Try it today!

Preparation time: 10 minutes **Cooking time:** 5 minutes **Servings:** 6

Ingredients:

1 tablespoon gelatin

¼ cup warm water

14 ounces canned coconut milk

14 ounces canned pumpkin puree

A pinch of salt

2 teaspoons vanilla extract

1 teaspoon cinnamon powder

1 teaspoon pumpkin pie spice

8 scoops stevia

3 tablespoons erythritol

Directions:

1. In a pot, mix pumpkin puree with coconut milk, a pinch of salt, vanilla extract, cinnamon powder, stevia, erythritol and pumpkin pie spice, stir well and heat up for a couple of minutes.

2. In a bowl, mix gelatin and water and stir.

3. Combine the 2 mixtures, stir well, divide custard into ramekins and leave aside to cool down.

4. Keep in the fridge until you serve it.

Enjoy!

Nutrition: calories 200, fat 2, fiber 1, carbs 3, protein 5

No Bake Cookies

These are stunning and so yummy!

Preparation time: 40 minutes **Cooking time:** 2 minutes **Servings:** 4

Ingredients:

1 cup swerve

¼ cup coconut milk

¼ cup coconut oil

2 tablespoons cocoa powder

1 and ¾ cup coconut, shredded

½ teaspoon vanilla extract

A pinch of salt

¾ cup almond butter

Directions:

1. Heat up a pan with the oil over medium high heat, add milk, cocoa powder and swerve, stir well for about 2 minutes and take off heat.

2. Add vanilla, a pinch of salt, coconut and almond butter and stir very well.

3. Place spoonful of this mix on a lined baking sheet, keep in the fridge for 30 minutes and then serve them.

Enjoy!

Nutrition: calories 150, fat 2, fiber 1, carbs 3, protein 6

Butter Delight

It not just tasty! It also looks amazing!

Preparation time: 10 minutes **Cooking time:** 4 minutes **Servings:** 16

Ingredients:

4 ounces coconut butter

4 ounces cocoa butter

¼ cup swerve

½ cup peanut butter

4 ounces dark chocolate, sugar free

½ teaspoon vanilla extract

1/8 teaspoon xanthan gum

Directions:

1. Put all butter and swerve in a pan and heat up over medium heat.

2. Stir until they all combine and then mix with xanthan gum and vanilla extract.

3. Stir well again, pour into a lined baking sheet and spread well.

4. Keep this in the fridge for 10 minutes.

5. Heat up a pan with water over medium high heat and bring to a simmer.

6. Add a bowl on top of the pan and add chocolate to the bowl.

7. Stir until it melts and drizzle this over butter mix.

8. Keep in the fridge until everything is firm, cut into 16 pieces and serve.

Enjoy!

Nutrition: calories 176, fat 15, fiber 2, carbs 5, protein 3

Tasty Marshmallows

Did you know you can make the keto version at home?

Preparation time: 10 minutes **Cooking time:** 3 minutes **Servings:** 6

Ingredients:

2 tablespoons gelatin

12 scoops stevia

½ cup cold water

½ cup hot water

2 teaspoons vanilla extract

¾ cup erythritol

Directions:

1. In a bowl, mix gelatin with cold water, stir and leave aside for 5 minutes.

2. Put hot water in a pan, add erythritol and stevia and stir well.

3. Combine this with the gelatin mix, add vanilla extract and stir everything well.

4. Beat this using a mixer and pour into a baking pan.

5. Leave aside in the fridge until it sets, then cut into pieces and serve.

Enjoy!

Nutrition: calories 140, fat 2, fiber 1, carbs 2, protein 4

Delicious Tiramisu Pudding

Try a keto tiramisu pudding today!

Preparation time: 2 hours and 10 minutes **Cooking time:** 0 minutes
Servings:

1

Ingredients:

8 ounces cream cheese

16 ounces cottage cheese

2 tablespoons cocoa powder

1 teaspoon instant coffee

4 tablespoons almond milk

1 and ½ cup splenda

Directions:

1. In your food processor, mix cottage cheese with cream cheese, cocoa powder and coffee and blend very well.

2. Add splenda and almond milk, blend again and divide into dessert cups.

3. Keep in the fridge until you serve.

Enjoy!

Nutrition: calories 200, fat 2, fiber 2, carbs 5, protein 5

Summer Dessert Smoothie

It's easy and super refreshing! You can try it today!

Preparation time: 5 minutes **Cooking time:** 0 minutes **Servings:** 2

Ingredients:

½ cup coconut milk

1 and ½ cup avocado, pitted and peeled

2 tablespoons green tea powder

2 teaspoons lime zest

1 tablespoon coconut sugar

1 mango thinly sliced for serving

Directions:

1. In your smoothie maker, combine milk with avocado, green tea powder and lime zest and pulse well.

2. Add sugar, blend well, divide into 2 glasses and serve with mango slices on top.

Enjoy!

Nutrition: calories 87, fat 5, fiber 3, carbs 6, protein 8

Lemon Sorbet

You only need 3 ingredients tom make this cool and keto dessert!

Preparation time: 5 minutes **Cooking time:** 0 minutes **Servings:** 4

Ingredients:

4 cups ice

Stevia to the taste

1 lemon, peeled and roughly chopped

Directions :

1. In your blender, mix lemon piece with stevia and ice and blend until everything is combined.

2. Divide into glasses and serve very cold.

Enjoy!

Nutrition: calories 67, fat 0, fiber 0, carbs 1, protein 1

Simple Raspberry Popsicles

It can't get any easier than this! You basically only need one ingredients: raspberries!

Preparation time: 2 hours **Cooking time:** 10 minutes **Servings:** 4

Ingredients:

1 and ½ cups raspberries

2 cups water

Directions:

1. Put raspberries and water in a pan, bring to a boil and simmer for 10

minutes at a medium temperature.

2. Pour mix in an ice cube tray, stick popsicles sticks in each and chill in the freezer for 2 hours.

Enjoy!

Nutrition: calories 60, fat 0, fiber 0, carbs 0, protein 2

Cherry And Chia Jam

Your family will love this great keto dessert!

Preparation time: 15 minutes **Cooking time:** 12 minutes **Servings:** 22

Ingredients:

3 tablespoons chia seeds

2 and ½ cups cherries, pitted

½ teaspoon vanilla powder

Peel from ½ lemon, grated

¼ cup erythritol

10 drops stevia

1 cup water

Directions:

1. Put cherries and the water in a pot, add stevia, erythritol, vanilla powder, chia seeds and lemon peel, stir, bring to a simmer and cook for 12 minutes.

2. Take off heat and leave your jam aside for 15 minutes at least.

3. Serve cold.

Enjoy!

Nutrition: calories 60, fat 1, fiber 1, carbs 2, protein 0.5

CPSIA information can be obtained
at www.ICGtesting.com
Printed in the USA
BVHW051733040521
606416BV00014B/1898